The Root Cl the Center of Money, Fear, Weight and Survival.

Learn To Heal Yourself With Your Energy (The Healing Energy Series)

Mirtha Contreras

Complementary Healing Disclaimer

As with all complementary therapies, none of the treatments/therapies/techniques listed in this book are meant to be a substitute for proper medical diagnosis, treatment or care from your doctor. If you are taking medication prescribed by your doctor, do not stop taking it if you decide to take a complementary approach to your health. It is recommended that you consult with a licensed medical doctor or physician before acting upon any recommendation that is made in this book.

Please also note that a good Reiki practitioner will always advise you to seek medical help from your doctor if she/he finds a health issue which is not already being treated by the patient's doctor.

Table of Contents

FREE Bonus Offer – Chakra Balancing Meditation (Audio)

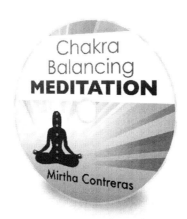

Thank you for downloading this book! It is my intention that it brings you the balance and healing you seek.

I have a special gift for you - an audio meditation you can download for FREE by visiting this web page:

http://OpenYourChakras.com/free-meditation

After you download the file, find a quiet spot and take a moment to close your eyes, relax, and follow along to this meditation. It will help to balance ALL your Chakras, clear them, and keep them aligned.

Enjoy!

I value your opinion. Please leave a review of this book on Amazon.com. Thank you!

Introduction

Chakras trouble may show up in many ways, shapes, and forms, but, as in dealing with most problems, to resolve these troubles we must begin at their roots. When it comes to Chakras and issues of energy flow, the Root Chakra – also known as the First Chakra – is the best place to start.

To protect ourselves from future energy imbalances, we must become aware of the importance the Root Chakra plays in absorbing our body's life energy and be mindful of the role it plays for all other Chakras. This awareness and practice will help us prevent future problems.

As you delve further into this book and discover the world of importance surrounding the Root Chakra, you may just find yourself waking up from a misspent life. When the First Chakra allows you to finally expand upon your energy reserves and really tap into the life energy of the world around you, you may feel better than ever before.

Of course, any progress will be short-lived if we aren't able to deliberately connect to our world – our environment, communities, and innermost selves – and stay connected. No reader will finish this book and go on to lead a life without future problems. Indeed, such troubles are a necessary part of life, but knowing what to do when they arise will allow us to make the most of what we've been handed here on Earth.

In fact, problematic situations have leant themselves to our evolution: as we respond to challenging situations in our physical environment over time, we slowly become the best possible being.

Evolutionary changes may take tens of thousands of years to become apparent, but that doesn't mean you can't have something of your own evolution right here, right now, in your own life.

Begin with this book – discover the importance of the Root Chakra, perform the exercises listed here, and uncover your own healing powers.

PART 1: Understanding Some Basic Concepts About Universal Life Energy and Our Energy Body

Even if this is a new idea for you, many cultures have studied and used the energy of their Chakras since ancient times. These techniques may have been called by many different names over thousands of years, but Chakra is the name for an energy vortex (which would look like a colored tornado funnel if you could see it) that connects your unique and true spirit to the spirit of all that is. It connects you, the individual, to the Universal Life Force Energy that flows eternally through space-time, and the Aura surrounding your body. This connection perfects us as conscious living beings. In this way, the physical body connects to the spiritual planes.

Hundreds of words have been used, spanning time and many cultures, to define our Life Force Energy. The roots of these words tell the story of how, across many cultures and planes of existence, beyond our physical being and Mother Earth, our energetic core connections have come to be recognized. Many study the Life Force Energy; some revere it.

In the 21st century, there is new recognition and hope that we will come to understand – and harness – these energetic birthrights. Humans continue to evolve, we now know, on levels beyond the physical. We have reached a time when the importance of the mind-body connection is understood and respected. If we take only a moment to open both the mind and heart before we look, see, hear, taste, and feel, our perception of the world will expand every time.

What Is Universal Life Force Energy?

Universal Life Force Energy is the vital and healing energy present in every living thing. This energy of life is known to many cultures by many different names: Chi, Prana, Pneuma, Ki, Orgone, Mana, Ruach, Baraka, Holy Ghost, and Bio-Plasmic Energy. You may have even heard The Beach Boys call it "good vibrations!"

The Universal Life Force Energy enters our body through the Aura surrounding our body, where it seeks and latches onto the Chakras. This continual energy flow, much like electricity, pours through us until something interrupts the process and a blockage develops. This could happen for several reasons, some which will be covered later in the book.

Anyone can rebalance their own Chakras through the use of visualization, color, sound, touch, or intention. Each Chakra exists on its own frequency and must be kept in tune. How do we do this? By tuning into the Universal Life Force Energy!

Our Energetic Body

The Chakras interact with the flow of Universal Life Force Energy by channeling it through our Aura. The Chakras and the Aura represent a few of the layers in our Energetic Body. Besides our Energetic Body, we have a Physical Body (comprised of our organs and physical systems), our Mental Body (made up of our thoughts) and our Emotional Body (which has to do with our emotions and feelings).

The state of our Aura as it interacts with the incoming Universal Life Force Energy can affect the quality of the energy that flows in and out of our being. Since we want a free flow of loving and healing energy, we must keep our Chakras in balance. That balance rewards us in many ways - giving us the ability to be happy, enjoy fulfilling relationships and prosperity, obtain mental clarity, live with purpose, be grounded, and possess a creative mind that is able to make dreams come true!

What Is the Aura?

An Aura is an Energetic Field that surrounds the human body. Everyone has an Aura. To most people, it is invisible, though they can experience it as a need to protect their "personal space." To those who can see it, the Aura appears as a transparent oval balloon large enough to easily surround the body with seven layers of subtle energy. Layer after layer, you are nestled in the very center. These layers connect and filter the energy of the cosmos - all that is- through our mind and body, making that energy accessible to our human senses when we are open to it.

The Aura expands and contracts as everyday life affects us. Those who know to look can see our emotions and reactions to everyday events within our Aura. Healers may comment that a person's Aura is shining, rich in one color, or displaying rainbows. Conversely, it could be muddy or dark, full of holes or gaps. The shape of the Aura could be malformed.

If someone is insisting that your Aura has issues, it's important to consider the source. There are well-meaning people who do some Aura reading as a hobby but, although they may be sympathetic, they have not been trained as a clear channel. If they lack this knowledge and ability, they may project their own imbalances and issues onto the person they believe they are "reading." In this case, it can happen that what the person actually describes is their own Aura as all of us must look through own Aura to see anything, including another person's body.

What Exactly Is a Chakra? Is It The Same Thing as Our Aura?

What Is a Chakra? What Do Chakras Do?

Historically, the word Chakra comes from the Sanskrit meaning "circle of life." A Chakra is a funnel-shaped energy vortex that channels vital energy - a concept explained earlier - to our physical body. That energy arrives by piercing and interacting with our Aura but also remains separate from it.

Very simply, the Chakras provide the necessary connection between vital energy and our spirit, or "self."

We know our physical bodies are capable of life without consciousness where, sadly, all personality and "real life" is absent. When we are suffering from illness or anxiety, our Chakras are imbalanced. If our energy centers become blocked and healing energies cannot flow freely, our physical bodies can suffer the consequences.

On the other hand, consciously utilizing our active Chakras can create the best possible life.

Chakras can also interact amongst each other to allow us to fully express our human potential as we pursue our dreams.

Each Chakra, or energy center, resonates at a specific vibrational frequency and is the key point of study in vibrational healing or medicine.

What's the Difference Between The Chakras and The Aura?

There is a distinct difference between Auras and Chakras. The Aura is an overall field surrounding the body. A Chakra is a distinct energy point within the body. Further, an Aura acts as a filter; its function is more subtle and less direct. A Chakra acts upon making an energetic connection, and that action depends on the strength of the incoming energy as much as the "openness" of the Chakra itself.

Both interact with each other, and both have the ability to effect change upon or balance one another.

How Many Chakras Do We Have? Where Are They Located?

Various cultures make varying claims about how many Chakras each of us have in our body. Some claim there are more than 100. The Hindu culture teaches that each of us contains twenty-one minor and seven major Chakras. The Chinese consider each of the many Meridians accessed through acupuncture to hold Chakras, numbering minor Chakras in the hundreds of thousands. That's a lot of needles!

In this book series, we're investigating the seven major Chakras recognized by every culture:

The First Chakra: Root (red)
The Second Chakra: Sacral or Splenic (orange)
The Third Chakra: Solar Plexus (yellow)
The Fourth Chakra: Heart (green)

The Fifth Chakra: Throat (blue)

The Sixth Chakra: Brow or Third Eye (indigo)

The Seventh Chakra: Crown (purple)

These energy vortices are numbered by counting up from the bottom, or the base of the spine, at the Root Chakra.

The Root Chakra is alone at the base of the spine, as is the Crown Chakra at the top center of your head – where the fontanel was open at birth to allow the skull to expand as one grew through infancy. These two Chakras sit at each end of the spinal cord, completing the connection of all Chakras within the body and ultimately providing a field of awareness that encompasses all our physical being.

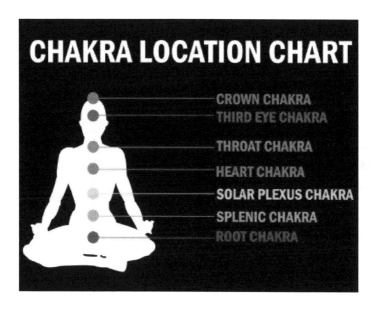

For a color version of this chart, which will help see each of the different colors of the chakras, please visit:

http://OpenYourChakras.com/ChakraLocationChart

The result is a bio-energetic sensory apparatus surrounding and woven into the human shell. Visualize them in the color frequency of each Chakra. Draw or paint them with their vibrant colors. We are living rainbows if we choose to see it.

You can read more about each of the different Chakras in the Appendix.

What Happens When Our Chakras Are Out of Balance?

You're living life as usual. Things are good - really humming along. Your step is so light and your outlook so rosy that people ask: "What's up with you? How can I get some of that?"

You know your mental state has been happy and clear for weeks. You feel fabulous. You not only ran a mile faster than usual, but you landed your best time. At work, you feel a substantial drive to succeed. You read a book about keeping your Chakras clear and tried a few of the ideas. Looks like it's working.

Right now, your Chakras are in balance. Naturally, you've noticed and chosen to maintain the gains you've made and the benefits that go along with them.

As the day proceeds, your boss, who had a recent fight with his wife and unconsciously wants to take it out on someone, calls you over. He raises his voice and you begin to feel anxious (First Chakra.). However, you're doing your job, meeting all your deadlines - you're even ahead of schedule on the next one.

He moves toward your desk and begins to berate you about a deadline that you've already met. He doesn't give you a second to say "It's already done." The words are stuck in your throat (Fifth Chakra).

As your boss walks away, you realize he's going to blame you for a problem that doesn't exist. You have a strong feeling in your gut that you're in trouble (Second Chakra). You decide to go home and work from there, where nothing more can happen to upset you.

However, before you can leave, the situation gets even worse. Your boss's boss shows up for a surprise visit. She speaks to your boss, who looks over at you, then quickly away. You feel as though someone punched you in the stomach – hard (Third Chakra). Now you're depressed because you've heard layoffs are definitely coming. The bosses didn't look at anyone but you. Your boss obviously thinks you're goofing off and missing important deadlines.

At this point, your First, Second, and Third Chakras, in quick succession, have been thrown out of balance at work, the place you depend upon for security.

You elect to go home with a tattered self-image (Fourth Chakra.) Your imagination takes off, dreaming up a myriad of awful things in store for you (Sixth Chakra). You assume you're getting the axe and bitterly think about the deadbeats who work in neighboring cubicles and how they should be fired in your stead.

When you arrive home, you're still so upset you feel nauseous. Even the comfort of home doesn't calm you.

Once again, you recall that Chakra book and its talk about Mindfulness. You remember how it explained that energy vibrates throughout our bodies, affecting the way we live our daily lives. There was a picture, wasn't there? You run off and retrieve the book.

Within minutes, you are looking at a drawing of a human body, with the bright colors of the Chakras lining up in a row down the center of the torso. You're a little nervous but you have nothing to lose.

You visualize your body with the colors down the center, just like in the picture, feeling all Chakras, from the First Chakra at the base of your spine to the Seventh Chakra at the top of your head. Silently, you breathe slowly and deeply and will the colors to balance you. After a while, you feel very calm -enough to make you stop worrying.

Today was just a tense day at work and you're happy you didn't react to the fear you felt earlier. You are reminded of the permanence of our true nature and that, as far as the incident at work goes, "this, too, shall pass."

PART 2: The Root Chakra - Your Power for Thriving and Surviving

What is the Root Chakra? Why Is It Important?

The existence of energy is a cosmic truth. The uses of energy are unending because energy cannot be created or destroyed – it simply changes form or flow. Creation energy, entering through the First Chakra, the Root, is called Kundalini energy, and is our life force.

The name given to the First Chakra, *Muladhara*, translates as "root support" or "support for the Kundalini." This shows its connection to its name in English, Root Chakra, and the energy it carries - the powerful Kundalini energy, which springs from Mother Earth and spirals through us from the time of our birth until we die.

The *Base* or *Root* Chakra can be found at the perineum, between the anus and the genitals. It vibrates at a low frequency to the musical note C and has a deep red color.

Muladhara, appropriately, is the only Chakra whose symbol points downward, toward the earth. This is a critical directional signal; its major purpose is our very survival and it represents our connection to the physical body we inhabit. The mere presence of the Muladhara suggests that we must survive as physical beings in this world in which we've been rooted.

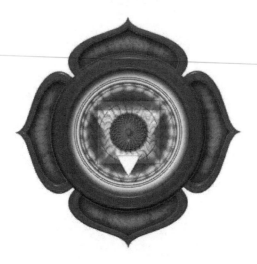

To view this image of the Muladhara in full color (beautiful!), please visit:

http://OpenYourChakras.com/Muladhara

The quantity and quality of the Kundalini energy channeled and moved by the First Chakra generates our will to live as well as the quality of our vitality. Our abilities to exist wholly in our world, as complete beings, and to reach our full potential as individuals depend upon a sustained flow of Kundalini energy.

For this reason, balancing all Chakras -and most especially the Root Chakra - ensures your full potential and quality of life as you move through each day.

The First Chakra is related to your senses of security, safety, and belonging. Your will to live, vitality, and essential physical functions also depend upon it, which is why the health of your First Chakra is so deeply connected to your spending habits, body weight, fears, and drive to succeed.

When this Chakra is at its optimal energetic frequency, it facilitates our connection to our inner power. We are then able to trust in Mother Earth, our local communities, and our own individual drive to provide what is necessary not only survive, but to *thrive*. We don't worry, we don't stress - we trust the universe, believe in our own promise, and feel that we are in the good hands of Mother Earth.

Because of the energy flow it provides, the First Chakra is essential to our existence. But it also rules how we perceive our self and all situations.. If the First Chakra is working as a clear, open, and perfect channel, it strengthens the "charge" of the energy that then flows up, through all the other Chakras.

As above, so below – or so the saying goes. Even when our higher Chakras are more finely tuned than the Root Chakra, they utterly depend on its balance. A stifled First Chakra will muddy the quality of energy flowing up the column. Muddied energy, filled with negative emotion of any description, can flow in place of positive, life-affirming energy.

Because each of the seven major Chakras controls or is related to various functions of the body, we must recognize that the Root Chakra affects every Chakra. Ultimately, through that influence and because it is the source of the life force energy, each Chakra depends on the condition and balance of the First Chakra, Muladhara.

How Can You Tell If Your Root Chakra Is Unbalanced?

If you think your Chakras are imbalanced, you absolutely must make sure that this imbalance doesn't begin with the First Chakra. Choose another Chakra to pick on! All kidding aside, truth can be found even in jokes, so read on to discover the symptoms and subsequent issues of an unbalanced or blocked Chakra.

An out-of-balance Root Chakra could express its condition with issues such as a lack of grounding, fear of moving forward in life, general anxiety, impatience, and addiction.

Physically, the body might respond with pain, growth problems, weight issues, colitis, diarrhea, hemorrhoids, or menopausal symptoms. You may also constantly lack energy, feel tired or, if your Root Chakra is overly active, you can be high-strung, have difficulty sleeping, or act aggressive and greedy.

Physical symptoms of an imbalance can manifest in the glands or organs nearest to or influenced by the First Chakra, including the spine, which may lead to scoliosis, back problems, or poor posture. Your feet, legs and hips may also suffer since they literally "ground" you and act as your body's foundation. Often a blocked Root Chakra results in problems with the reproductive organs such as the ovaries, prostate, cervix, and testicles. This blocked energy is also commonly responsible for blood deficiencies, constipation, and bladder infections.

Other common signs of a blocked or stressed Root Chakra are sexual debility and low libido. Sexual activity requires a great deal of energy from the body, so when your body is struggling to heal itself, it lowers your sexual desire in order to conserve your energy for healing. If the Root Chakra is overactive, then the person may become sexually addicted. When this occurs, sex is no longer an act of pleasure and enjoyment, but instead becomes a source of pain.

On the emotional level, someone with a blocked Root Chakra experiences temper tantrums; repressed anger explodes outwards due to the immense strain of containing it inside for so long.

Mentally, you tend to experience a deep sense of angst as your mind fills with dread and excessive fear about the future. You may also feel mentally spacey, worry too much, or behave in an overly cautious manner without need. You may also have a tendency to dwell on situations that occurred in the past, unable to let things go.

When your Root Chakra is unbalanced you are poorly grounded and your spatial understanding is impaired. You may stumble around physically, mentally, spiritually, and emotionally. Grounding enhances your ability to function effectively on a day-to-day basis. You may have trouble with your finances and with how you relate to others in your community. Also, when we do not feel some connection to the Earth, we lack a general appreciation of nature.

An Over-Active Root Chakra Exhausts You from the Inside Out

Physically, an overactive Root Chakra leads to difficulty in gaining weight, a low tolerance for cold environments, and a low immune system that causes you to get sick easily and often. Your body may often feel restless and drive you into days full of exhausting activity.

Mentally, you struggle because you want to get a million things done, but it's difficult to focus on anything. Your thought flow seems to suffer from countless interruptions. You encounter strong desires to accumulate excessive wealth and dominate as many competitors as possible. Often you take actions before considering the consequences, and this recklessness gets you into trouble. You find it very difficult to trust others.

Emotionally, you are prone to aggressive behavior and often experience abnormal, excessive sexual desires. It becomes very difficult to understand anyone else's point of view, and your emotions become hard to control. You find yourself obsessed with money, work, and material displays of success.

The hyperactive Root Chakra commonly manifests as a series of passionate relationships that end quickly, projects that you start with great enthusiasm but don't finish, a mishandling of your finances, and regular power struggles with work colleagues.

Other Signs of a Weak Root Chakra

Physically, a depleted Root Chakra can result in trouble losing weight and a weakened sex drive, causing impotence in men and frigidity in women. Eating disorders often develop as well. Candida overgrowth and lower back pain are often chronic issues, bowel movements are irregular or difficult, and there is an overall lack of energy in all areas of life. You generally feel clumsy and awkward in social situations, and you lack self-confidence.

Mentally, you cannot get anything done on time or plan things well because you lack focus and fall victim to inaction. Every goal seems difficult to accomplish. You find yourself giving up on projects easily, and you may even contemplate suicide.

Emotionally, you feel a general lack of enthusiasm in your life, which may lead to depression. It seems like you never have enough money for life's necessities, and you struggle to make ends meet. You convince yourself that people are against you even when they are not. You lack the support and strength to achieve your goals. When people challenge you, often you choose to take the easy way out and let others get what they want; this behavior leads to allowing others to habitually walk all over you. One manifestation may be a dead-end relationship that you want to end but can't find the courage. Repeatedly you experience various circumstances in which you become the victim. Even when you make plans, they become difficult to follow and usually fall apart, often leaving you with the feeling that your life is going in useless circles.

Other Signs of a Root Chakra Imbalance

The First Chakra also governs your cultural roots and foundations, especially your early home life. If you had a difficult childhood, balance in this Chakra may have always been a challenge to maintain, especially if you were completely unaware of it. Imbalance may have been expressed as sensory issues that led to learning disabilities. Such disabilities can survive or recur in adulthood until you recognize the issue and consciously resolve it. If you often find yourself fighting with siblings over childhood events or complaining to others of what you did not receive growing up, this could be a sign you need to focus on this issue and bring it into balance. Being unable to move on from the past -or out of one phase and into the next - is typical behavior resulting from an imbalanced First Chakra.

Our First Chakra binds us to the Earth and gives us a sense of place, home, and security. Given the strong and grounded nature of this Chakra, any indication of feeling spacey, off-centered, detached, or disconnected from your family and close friends signals a possible imbalance.

28

The silver lining here is that when our Root Chakra is in balance, we have access to our fullest capabilities at all levels: our perceptions are clear and real, and our ability to ascertain our true needs and make judgments free of fear is strong.

How Can I Ascertain the Condition of My Root Chakra?

If you would like further clarification and advice about the health of your Root Chakra, seek the professional opinion of an experienced energy healer. These professionals are great resources in helping you to determine if your Root Chakra is blocked, hyperactive or lacking energy.

Psychic healers, pranic healers, Reiki healers, Ayurvedic doctors, and similar therapists can detect your Chakra health through the use of pendulums and their expert intuition and training. Gifted spiritual counselors can actually see your Chakra activity reflected in the subtle Aura around your body.

What Can Cause Your Root Chakra to Become Blocked?

Generally, blockage begins when our emotions and needs are repressed or not met. We have infinite potential to adapt to drastic life situations, but sometimes a bad situation can cause one or more of the Chakras to shut down temporarily as part of a survival mechanism.

Root Chakra blockage stops the flow of Kundalini Energy, our life force. An open, balanced Root Chakra provides a wide-open gateway for life force energy, maximizing our energy potential. Again, all other Chakras depend on a strong universal life force flow at the Root Chakra. The life force energy that enters at the Root Chakra must be of sufficient quality and quantity to rise up the spine, spiraling to the other six major Chakras and beyond.

As with most problems, a Chakra imbalance can start small - as a minor imbalance, such as a lack of confidence in yourself and life in general (a deficiency of energy imbalance), or permitting and engaging in domineering behavior (an excessive energy imbalance). You might have trouble setting goals or achieving the goals you've set. When an imbalance goes unnoticed - or worse, ignored - the intensity of the problem worsens. When an imbalance builds over a long period of time, it can result in complete blockage of the Root Chakra.

Many different things can cause blocks in our Root Chakras, and here are some of the most common causes:

Certain Types of Surgery

- **Cesarean section surgery** can lead to major Root Chakra blockages because of the subtle, physical traumas involved in this operation. Particularly when this operation is performed suddenly, in emergency circumstances, and the mother has not had time to sufficiently prepare herself psychologically and emotionally, then the body experiences this surgery as a much more traumatic operation.

Such a trauma is often stored as energy in the Root Chakra, even after the procedure, and often women report feeling the side effects of a C-section for months afterward - sometimes longer.

A woman's body spends a great deal of time preparing for delivery, so when the delivery does not happen naturally through the birth canal, it takes time for the body to accept that the child is no longer in the uterus.

A great deal of energy builds up around the Root Chakra in preparation for a natural birth, which isn't properly released during a C-section. This energy sits stagnate for a long time, contributing to possible Root Chakra imbalances, such as postpartum depression. Some of these mothers describe dreaming that they are still about to go to the hospital to deliver their child for weeks after they've already had their baby. On a subtle level, this Root Chakra obstruction is partially due to a lack of completion in the birthing process.

- **Abdominal surgery**, like an appendectomy or operations on the stomach, kidney, and liver, also contributes to Root Chakra blockages for various reasons. Surgeries of this nature are often critical in saving a patient's life, and, like any other potentially fatal circumstance, these surgeries put a great strain on the Root Chakra, which controls our survival instincts.

The Root Chakra blockages that occur after these surgeries also help to explain some of the common post-operation side effects. For example, since the Root Chakra is responsible for the energetic and physical elimination processes of your body, a blockage here can lead to short-term bowel paralysis.

Those who don't take sufficient rest after an abdominal or other critical surgery may suffer from greater Root Chakra damage as a result; this complication is due to added stress on the Root Chakra as the body is forced to repair damaged tissues without much needed rest.

Traumatic Circumstances Surrounding Your Birth and Childhood

Things that happened at the time of your birth and throughout your childhood have lasting effects on your Root Chakra because of the increased sensitivity and vulnerability that surrounds babies and children. Some events may have lasting effects on your sense of security.

- Doctors in the growing field of prenatal and perinatal psychology are finding that if **your birth was traumatic**, you may develop recurring behaviors and emotions later in life reflecting that experience. A baby's earliest experiences are sometimes stored in the Root Chakra, leading to long-lasting energy blockage. For example, an obsessive desire for control can stem from your experience of being delivered with forceps. Similarly, if your mother's labor was induced, then you may go on to resent interruptions and external attempts to control you in any way.

- **Failure to bond with your mother** creates a block in your Root Chakra because it leads to feelings of insecurity and instability early in life. To newborns and infants, the mother figure is the foundation of their entire world. Any absence of maternal bonding instills early apprehensions about your personal security and forces you to feel you must fend for yourself.

- **Childhood trauma** severely triggers the fight-or-flight response in your Root Chakra. Since children can't defend themselves in dangerous or frightening situations, they may develop deep resentments, fears, and even desires for revenge that manifest later in life as the results of Root Chakra damage. It can take people a long time to consciously recognize these stagnant, trapped emotions and release them.

- An **excessively strict upbringing** often leads to lasting Root Chakra obstructions as children become adults. When children are harshly punished at a young age - particularly when the punishment is a form of physical abuse - their Root Chakra trauma leaves them unable to appropriately defend themselves as adults. If you had such an experience, you may have great difficulty making decisions that are in your own best interest because you fear the disapproval of others. A healthy Root Chakra empowers you to feel confident about the choices you make and take care of your own needs, but the blockage resulting from an overly strict upbringing prevents you from doing these things effectively.

- **Radical religious views** have a great impact on your Root Chakra. Ideally, your religious views serve as a source of inner strength; they provide you with feelings of security, purpose, and value as a human being. If a child is raised in a religious environment that advocates anger or the use of violence as forms of training or worship, their survival instincts may become drastically impaired or even hyperactive. When this happens, this intense energy is trapped in the Root Chakra like a poison.

The Absence of Healthy Relationships

A lack of connection with your community disempowers your Root Chakra and contributes to blockages. Extreme isolation and behaviors that separate you from other people in your environment encourage irrational fears to flourish and take over the mind. To heal conditions like these, it's crucial to unblock the Root Chakra in order to allow healthy connections with others to form again.

What Causes Minor Root Chakra Blockages?

Since some of the Root Chakra's main functions involve conserving energy reserves and eliminating superfluous negative energies from our systems, anything that interrupts the body's natural flow of elimination can also lead to a Root Chakra blockage. Remember that a healthy, balanced diet and a harmonious, environmentally-friendly lifestyle are fundamental parts of any healing process to restore balance in your Root Chakra.

Balance Your Root Chakra with these Simple Techniques

Throughout life, each and any of our Chakras can move in and out of balance. By using mindfulness and keeping your perceptions clear and focused, you will quickly notice any signs of imbalance. Using these same qualities - mindfulness and clarity - can quickly restore you to balance.

Fostering Chakra awareness can alert you to the earliest stages of an imbalance, helping you to identify and remedy the problem at the start. Immediately correcting an imbalance will keep it from intensifying, moving to other Chakras, and eventually becoming a blockage. If a blockage does occur, the longer you have allowed yourself to remain unaware of it - or worse, have been conscious of it but did not act to correct it - the more effort and energy will be required to clear it.

If you maintain a state of mindfulness as part of your everyday awareness, small imbalances are easily reframed or reversed and a blockage is unlikely to occur.

Earlier in the book, we explored how certain energies help activate and recharge the First Chakra to improve our lives. Now I'd like to invite you to do a few of these fun techniques that will empower you to flow through life as pleasantly as possible. These exercises will show you how to reinvent yourself and rediscover love, helping you to create the best possible life for yourself. .

Notice that you've been invited to partake in these activities – not ordered. These exercises are not a job that you must complete – nor are they a forced experiment. By approaching these techniques with a negative attitude, you would forgo the key to their success..

Do these activities for yourself, on your own, as part of your initiative to create your personal transformation. Use this time to take care of yourself and remember that, even when things aren't going as planned, it's important to be able to access your inner support system.

Remember that life is about more than constantly traveling toward a goal; it's often during our travels that we do much of our learning and growing. While it is very important to recognize when something is wrong in your life, it's equally important for you to act on this realization! Realize that a negative situation can function as a catalyst to inspire you to begin your transformation. Do these exercises anytime you're feeling scattered or unfocused and they will help you regain clarity.

Technique #1:
Reduce Your Fears to Ashes

We all face different fears every day. Thankfully, there are many easy ways to conquer even the biggest fears.

This written exercise that you can do in your spare time, or whenever you feel your confidence is waning, can help you alleviate such fears. Performing this technique will allow you to become aware of your fears before finally letting them go.

In order to complete this exercise, it's important to sit down somewhere quiet, where you can really focus on yourself and your inner feelings related to your fear.

Take a few deep breaths before starting. Doing so will help you begin to focus, clearing your mind of all other life distractions. For the moment, forget about your job, kids, bills, and any other stress factors. During this exercise, all those things must be put on the back burner while you focus on the beliefs that are holding you back. Eliminate any distractions: don'tsit in front of the computer so you won't be tempted to surf or check your Facebook, don't have the TV on in the background, and put your cell phone in silent mode. Rather, think to yourself, "This is 'me' time."

This simple but wonderful exercise will help you become aware of any fears preventing you from realizing your dreams and to subsequently release them.

To begin, take a sheet of paper and think about a dream, goal, or project you want to achieve. Next, make a list of everything you fear will prevent you from realizing that dream or goal. For example, write something like this:

I, [your name], am afraid that I will not be able to accomplish (project or goal) because…

Write down everything you see as an obstacle. Remember that this list is for your eyes only, so it's okay to really dive in and even over-think it a bit. This way, you'll be sure to cover every aspect of your fears. Allow yourself to really get in touch to your inner fears and beliefs. Nobody is watching.

Here is an example:

I, Susan Blake, am afraid that I will not be able to get a new car because…

I won't be able to save enough money

I won't be approved for a car loan

I won't have anywhere to park it

It might get stolen

I only drive automatic

After you write down every imaginable fear, read your list aloud. What this does is remove these "fear factors" from you. They now exist only on the paper before you.

Next, notice how each of these fears makes you feel. How do they affect your body? By going through this process, you are openly exposing yourself to each fear as a whole, a very popular method of healing.

Now burn the list.

As the list burns, you'll feel your confidence building. This simple action proves that these fears have no control over you. The only person in control of your life is you. As this realization sinks in, you'll feel driven to take the necessary action steps to turn your project or dream into a reality.

Remember that your fears and limiting beliefs are your only true obstacles in life. Realize that someone, somewhere, overcame each of the fears holding you back. Just as others surpassed those same fears, so shall you. This is how people reach their full potential in life and many dreams are realized.

Technique #2:
Connect with Your Conscious Awareness

When you get out of bed in the morning, pull out a blank sheet of paper and pen. Take three long, deep breaths and write down any three events, people, or recurring situations that you'd like to let go of forever. They should come to you easily as they are the things that are holding you back by keeping you trapped in old memories of the past.

As you go through your daily routine, take a little time to connect with these three things thinking about what each has taught you. Think about the lessons acquired by your dealings with these people or situations. Become aware that now that you have learned these lessons you can now let go of this limiting belief or fear. You no longer need to bear the weight of that experience any longer or continue to feel guilt.

Before you release the three things you've chosen for elimination, give mental thanks to each one for the things it has taught you and, without feeling any attachment, just let them go.

At the end of the day, take a long bath and imagine the water helping to cleanse your spirit as you cultivate grateful feelings for being able to move on.

Becoming aware of this excess baggage and consciously releasing it helps you close its cycle helping you get ready to start a healthy new cycle.

Before you go to bed, take the list of three people or things and burn it. Doing so will symbolize the final purification and release of these three weights, burdens that you don't need to worry about anymore.

When you wake up the following morning, get another piece of paper and a pen. Take three long, deep breaths and write down three things that you wish to create in your life - dreams that you want to make a reality.

Take a few minutes and imagine what it would be like to experience those things now. Think about it in great detail and trying to involve all of your senses. As you visualize, thank those goals for coming true with a heart full of infinite gratitude.

Keep this special sheet of paper with you and repeat this visualization each morning until you finally achieve these dreams.

This powerful exercise strengthens your focus, adding to your odds of prosperity, improving your wellbeing, and reaching the goals that are most important to you. Over time, you'll reconnect with your own inner power to fulfill your ultimate potential.

Technique #3:
To Be, to Do and to Have

This activity trains you to reconnect with your inner strengths and focus on what really fulfills you. It will allow you to easily develop a steady focus on your goals and access 100 percent of your energy in your daily life. Performing this technique can result in a plethora of benefits: wealth, overall prosperity, and a deeper appreciation for all of your potential.

Starting now, you have a new opportunity to look into the future. Where are you going in life? What do you really like, and what do you really want to do? Consider your talents and remember where others have told you your talents lie. When and where do you feel as comfortable as a fish swimming in water?

Begin the process by taking three deep breaths, and, on a new piece of paper, write ten things that you like about yourself. List absolutely any aspect of yourself, and the inventory you create will help you clarify your strengths. You need not write a book - for example, you could list things like, "I'm a good student," "I pay attention to detail," or "I'm friendly."

Continue the exercise by writing down five things that you love to do. You can make them general or specific - for example, you could just use the word "cooking" or delve into more details if you like.

Next, create another list of five things that you wish you had Dream as big as you wish - a car or your own business - the important point is to consider what really gets you excited.

Let's take another look at this exercise by putting it into practice.

Pick three things that you like most about yourself, two things you love to do, and two things that you really wish you had. How do you choose these things? As you read the list, pay attention to what really gets you excited. Pay attention to the feelings and sensations in your body as you create these lists. Choose a combination that makes sense for you and the life you want to live.

There. You have figured out your purpose in life!

For example, if you chose personal traits like being physically fit, communicative, and creative, then you can combine them with fun activities you wrote like cooking and writing. Add to that the wish to have your own business, and you have several great possibilities:

1) You can open your own restaurant.

2) You can write a cookbook.

3) You can make new food products or delicacies and sell them to restaurants.

Now go on and make your dreams come true!

Technique #4:
Root Chakra Healing Visualization

This helpful visualization exercise will revitalize your Root Chakra by consciously redirecting the natural energy flow within your body. This simple technique allows you to receive more natural, healing energy from the universe.

Begin by sitting in a comfortable, relaxed posture and closing your eyes. Now imagine a large, beautiful tree in front of you. It's strong and full of vibrant green leaves that spread out in all directions. Its thick roots spread and sink far below the earth's surface. These roots form a firm foundation and create a lifelong bond between the tree and the entire planet.

Just like this tree, visualize that your body has roots of its own and that they extend downwards to penetrate deep inside the planet, spreading out in all directions below the ground's surface. Your long, thick roots are moving out from the base of your spine as they stretch further underground. These new roots of yours are allowing you to absorb the positive, healing energy of Mother Earth, drawing it up into your body. Feel the living energy of the Earth traveling up through your roots.

This refreshing water symbolizes perfect love, and it contains the power necessary to restore your balance. As your roots drink the pure energy of unconditional love, you feel a new, healing awareness within you. You allow yourself to absorb this profound love up through your roots, into your spine and throughout your body. You are complete and deeply satisfied with this infinite reserve of energy. Thank Mother Earth for everything she is freely giving you and slowly begin to lift your roots out of the ground until they fully merge into your body. Know that your connection with Mother Earth is eternal, and gradually open your eyes again.

Now that you've connected with your ultimate energy source, you're refreshed and ready to face life's challenges once again. Practice this visualization for as long as you wish, wherever you wish. For best results, try doing this while seated outside, underneath a tree.

Technique #5:
Your Treasure Map

This exercise is also known as a dream or vision board, and it works by directing our thoughts to consistently flow towards our goals. Our thoughts carry the power to attract what we're seeking and bring it to fruition. Thoughts become beliefs, and beliefs focus our actions to match our priorities.

A focused mind gives you the energy needed to accomplish your life projects with 100 percent of your enthusiasm, allowing you to enjoy every step of this process.

The map you'll create to your treasure chest of fulfilled wishes helps you connect with your inner power of manifesting. Therefore, it gives you the self-confidence you need to reach your goals. Every time you look at your treasure map, it reminds you of the hopes in your heart and inspires you to keep moving toward them.

Before You Begin

It's very important to address any fears and doubts you might have regarding your goals and dreams. To do this, use the Conscious Awareness technique explained in the previous section. You should express them, write them down on paper, and burn them to purify your mind of these limiting thoughts, so that they don't prevent you from materializing the goal on your personal treasure map.

The next step in this process is to clarify exactly what it is you want.

Start by taking three full breaths and then begin writing a list of what you would like to manifest right now. Organize this list by putting the things that are the most important to you at the top. When your most important goal becomes clear, focus on this one first.

When we try to accomplish more than one goal at a time, our energy becomes scattered, and that's exactly what we're trying to avoid. We want to conserve and direct our strength toward one project at a time, making it easier to achieve. After the first project is complete, you can always come back to this list and begin the next project.

Make sure that your treasure map of dreams is your own personal project. Do not make a treasure map for someone else because it only works when people make their own. To clarify, you can seek to manifest a loving relationship in general, but you can't manifest a relationship that violates another person's free will. Making a map for your child also crosses the boundaries of free will; children should make their own maps. If you have a common goal with your partner to get a new house, however, you can make a map together because both of you are actively involved in making this dream happen.

What Materials Do You Need?

- Choose a large piece of cardboard or a sheet of paper in your favorite color.
- Select colored markers, paints or any other colorful arts supplies you like to use.
- Use a variety of magazines with pictures related to your dream or download and print pictures you find online.
- Set aside a few hours to have fun creating your treasure map because you are doing it for you!

Making Your Map

At the top, make a title for your map that clarifies what you're seeking. For example:

This is a healthy body for me
This is the apartment that I am open to receiving
This is the car I deserve
This is my perfect match

Make the title eye-catching by unleashing your creative imagination using cut-out letters or anything else you like.

You must create the necessary conditions to allow your treasure to come forth in a positive way. For example, let's say that your project is to manifest a new home. Besides doing your treasure map, you should begin to prepare your current home for its next occupants. Give it a good cleaning, fix what needs to be fixed before selling or renting, and take care of the necessary paperwork to make the transition easier. Also, write down all the reasons why you are grateful for having lived there. Literally thank your current home for giving you shelter and for the good experiences you had while living there.

Start acting as if you are about to get what you want. If you want a new car, for example, head to the car dealership and check out the car you want, research car insurance and loans, and so on. At the car dealership, sit in your future car and ask someone to take a picture of you with your camera. A photo of how happy you look seated in your dream car is the perfect central image for your treasure map!

If your goal is to heal your body, use a picture of a healthy organ on your map. Include pictures of happy, healthy people who are free of the illness you want to heal. You can add your own picture to help you visualize your healed self.

You can also add affirmations to the map that describe how you want the healing process to manifest. For example, write affirmations on the treasure map for your new home like this:

I'm grateful to live in a quiet and safe environment.
I appreciate having three spacious bedrooms.
I love the natural lighting in my new home.
My new neighbors are wonderful people; I love spending time with them.

Use illustrations to help you visualize what inspires grateful feelings.

Affirmations like these have worked very well for me in achieving my own goals. Make sure your affirmations are in the present tense; you are developing the mindset that you've already begun to receive your treasure, so you are already thankful for it. The more you stay in the mindset of asking for something, the more you remain in a state of mental poverty.

To complete your map, write this sentence at the bottom:

"All of this or something better is happening to me right now in perfect harmony with everyone else in the universe. Thank you, God [Universe, Higher Self, or whatever you envision as the Higher Power], because I know it's already coming my way!"

Where Should You Keep Your Treasure Map?

To track your progress on this journey to your goal, keep the map in a visible location so that you can continuously connect to your dream. It doesn't matter if anyone else sees it, but, if you prefer, you can keep it in a private place until it manifests. Remember that it's best not to put a time limit on your map or set a date to achieve your goal; trust the universe instead to know the perfect time for your project to materialize.

Once you reach the final treasure, celebrate! Express your gratitude and acknowledge your personal achievement.

If you create a map and later you realize that this treasure is not actually what you want, then you can simply destroy it and start fresh. If you created your map on something durable like a corkboard, then you only need to get rid of the images and everything else that you placed there; save the corkboard to use for your next treasure map!

More Techniques You Can Do on Your Own to Balance Your Root Chakra

Affirmations

Take a look at the following list of affirmations that are specially formulated to activate your Root Chakra. Pick one that you like and write it down. Memorize it. Meditate on it. Create Post-It notes and position them around your house where you'll see them often. Repeat your chosen mantra to yourself whenever you remember. After a week of repetition, pick a new affirmation and repeat the process.

I am safe and secure. I have what I need.
I trust the natural flow of life. I trust that my needs will be met.
I feel comfortable with my body.
I take responsibility for my life.
I am open to the best that life has to offer.
I make healthy choices.
I am divinely protected and guided.
I am open to new ideas, new thoughts, and new people to enhance my life.
Life is good.

Mudras

A *Mudra*, which is Sanskrit for "closure" or "seal," is a certain body position - mostly involving our hands and fingers - that influences out body's energy.

The following are some Mudras that you can use to open your Root Chakra. You could really do them anytime, but it's a good idea to use them while meditating, as they are generally more effective if done daily and maintained for at least fifteen minutes or so. Also, use both hands when possible, since the effect is stronger this way.

Prithvi Mudra

This is a good Mudra to help you increase stability and feel strong and confident. Touch the tip of your thumb with the tip of your ring finger. Keep the other fingers extended.

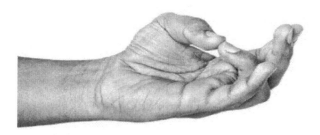

Pran Mudra

This is also known as the Life Mudra, since Prana, as discussed previously, is the Life Force Energy. Bring the tips of your little finger and ring finger to the tip of your thumb. Extend your other fingers.

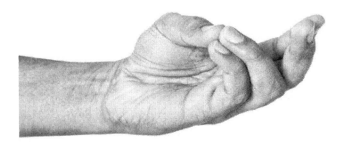

Surya Mudra

This is a good Mudra to use to help you lose weight and lower bad cholesterol. Bend your ring finger until it touches the base of your thumb. Place your thumb over the ring finger so that the tip of your thumb touches the second knuckle of your ring finger. Extend your other fingers.

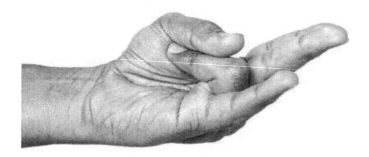

Mantras and Sounds

A Mantra is a sound, syllable, word or words that have the power to transform energy.

The musical note associated with the Root Chakra is C and the associated vowel is U, pronounced "uh" (as in cup).

Here are some Mantras that you can use to balance your Root Chakra:

Soham

This is Sanskrit for "I Am." You can mentally say "so" as you inhale and "ham" as you exhale.

Bija Mantra: "Lam"

"Bija" means seed. When you say a Bija Mantra out loud, the sound you make resonates with the energy that is related to the Chakra, helping to activate its energy. The Bija Mantra associated with the First Chakra is "Lam" (sounds like "lum").

Mul Mantra

Mul Mantra literally means "Root Mantra" and helps eliminate fear. It is a complex Mantra and it might be best to look for it online and listen to it as you meditate.

Ganesh Mantra

Lord Ganesh is a Hindu deity who represents the energy that helps us overcome all obstacles. He also rules the Muladhara

Chakra, which is why we include this Mantra here. A common Mantra used to ask Lord Ganesh for blessings is:

Om Gam Ganapataye Namaha

Make sure you listen to this Mantra online (on YouTube, for example) to be certain that sure you're saying it right!

You can chant these Mantras while concentrating on your Root Chakra, looking at a picture of the Root Chakra (see Part One of this book), or dancing and stomping your feet. Have fun with them!

Angelic Healing and Prayer

Seeking angelic healing and using prayer to repair your Root Chakra are both very helpful techniques to clear Root Chakra blockages. This therapeutic tool is suitable for anyone who has some quiet time and a little faith. You can use these techniques to enhance a crystal healing session, too.

Make yourself comfortable in a sitting or reclining position and dim the lights if possible. Place both of your hands on the sides of your lower abdomen, near the tops of your hip joints.

Close your eyes and allow yourself to fully relax with some slow, steady breaths for a few minutes. After your breathing becomes deep and calm, visualize your Root Chakra as a small red ball of light at the base of your spine. Mentally ask for the angels of the earth to come to you now; tell them that you want their help to heal you.

After a minute, visualize that an angel's soothing light begins to surround your Root Chakra and feel its loving, grounded energy supporting you. Energy from your own hands and the angel are now working together in harmony. If it helps, you can also visualize as many details as you wish about the angel's appearance during this healing. When you feel you are ready, thank the angel for supporting you and gradually let your visualizations fade away naturally before you open your eyes again.

Alternatively, you can use any prayer form of your choice to help repair your Root Chakra. What's important is to invoke assistance from a source of power greater than yourself and to remain open to the experience so you can receive healing. Be honest in your prayers and express yourself fully to the universe in order to help release the tensions trapped inside your Root Chakra.

Meditation is also a form of prayer through which you can ask for guidance and healing, and then just sit quietly to reflect and observe yourself without judgment.

Other Simple Ways to Balance Your Root Chakra

Maintain your Root Chakra balance or correct minor imbalances by following these other tips:

- Walk barefoot in your garden, on the grass at the park, or on a beach in the morning or after the sand has cooled.

- Enjoy some time in nature. Meditate (you can also do yoga, tai chi, or say your affirmations) under a tree, in your garden, or at the beach.

- If you are able to, run, jog, bicycle, or power walk to reduce stress and increase your physical vitality. Most sports (try martial arts!) are excellent for the Root Chakra.

- Any type of dancing (try belly dancing or flamenco!) or foot-stomping will help activate this Chakra and your connection to life.

- Do some gardening, take care of a plant, or plant a tree. This will help you connect with Mother Earth.

- Work with pottery or ceramics, or try sculpting.

- Take care of your feet - get a foot massage or a pedicure!

- Do some squats.

- Donate some money to charity.
- Learn more about your community and cultural values.

- Remember that red is the color of the Root Chakra. Wear some red clothes or accessories -have fun with red shoes or socks! - and place some red accents around your house.

- Be mindful of any thoughts of deficiency, such as "I don't have enough," "I'm not good enough," or "I can't afford it." The moment these thoughts arise, cut them out and replace them with an opposing, positive statement. Remember, negative thoughts only have power over you if give it to them.

- Do your Kegels! Exercising what's known as the "Kegel" muscles is another good way to strengthen your Root Chakra. Contract your muscles as if you were trying to control the flow of urine. Hold for three to five seconds, then relax those muscles. Imagine yourself receiving the abundance of the Earth as you relax the muscles and then send that energy up to your other Chakras as you contract them.

What Foods Can You Eat to Help Activate Your Root Chakra?

- Root vegetables, of course! Try carrots, potatoes, radishes, onions, turnips, peanuts, beets, and garlic.
- Eat some protein-rich foods, like meat and tuna, eggs, beans, peanut butter, and tofu and other soy products.
- You can also enjoy spices such as cinnamon, vanilla, paprika, and cayenne pepper for the benefit of your Root Chakra, as well as sesame seeds and saffron.
- Finally, remember to include red fruits and vegetables, such as strawberries, raspberries, watermelon, plums, cherries, pomegranates, tomatoes, red cabbage, radishes, beetroot, chilies, red pepper, and blood oranges. You can also drink guava or pink grapefruit juice.

An Overview of Advanced Techniques to Clear Your Root Chakra

There are many advanced healing techniques that are very effective in clearing and balancing your Root Chakra. Some require direct assistance from an experienced healer, but there are several that you can do by yourself in the comfort of your home. However, these usually require some special materials or knowledge. Please note that for any very severe Root Chakra damage, it's always advisable to seek personal guidance from a healer for best results.

Gemstone Therapy

Using crystals and gemstones is the safest way to begin energetically healing yourself without risk of side effects. These are safe for everyone to use. Crystals are capable of absorbing, emitting, conserving, and focusing electromagnetic energy, and they are especially beneficial in cleansing and transforming negative energies that block the Root Chakra.

Which Crystals Are Best for Healing the Root Chakra?

Any black- or red-colored crystals will help in this process. However, the following crystals are the most effective in healing the Root Chakra: garnet, ruby, smoky quartz, hematite, black tourmaline, bloodstone, obsidian, red jasper, carnelian, azurite, and chrysocolla. Sometimes, if the Root Chakra disturbance is causing symptoms of depression, you can also use citrine and golden-yellow topaz.

There are two simple ways to use crystals in Root Chakra healing - via crystal layouts or crystal elixirs.

Crystal Layouts

Crystal layouts are excellent for helping you to relax and easily absorb the natural, healing energy of the stones. To begin, cleanse your crystals of any subtle energy that they're carrying from the past. The quickest way to do this is by holding them under running water for about a minute with the clear intention that they are being completely purified. You can also soak them in homemade salt water or ocean water overnight - as long as they are not friable (easily crumbled) - and you can then let them dry in direct moonlight to fully recharge. If your crystals seem to lose some color during a soak, that can mean they are artificial, dyed crystals. Genuine red coral, for example, should not lose its color in water.

When your crystals are ready, prepare a quiet space where you can lay down without interruption. Lie down and place the crystals directly above and around your Root Chakra, near the pubic bone and on your hip joints. You can also place your feet slightly apart and position one crystal on the bed between your feet. Now close your eyes and mentally ask the universe to help heal you through these crystals.

After some time, it's normal to feel subtle movements of energy around your Root Chakra, but, if the Chakra is very blocked, you may not notice any sensations during your first session. You can remain relaxed like this for up to half an hour. Remember to cleanse your crystals once more afterwards.

More complex crystal layouts consist of arranging many crystals in geometric patterns around and on your body, and these specifically direct your body's energy flow in new directions for healing.

Crystal Elixirs

First, make sure to clean your crystals and check that they have no toxic properties when soaked in water. The crystals mentioned above are all safe to use for elixirs, but some crystals - like malachite, for example - become toxic when combined with water. Such crystals require special care and cleansing from other special crystals..

Place your crystals inside a glass jar filled with purified drinking water - spring or mineral water work well for elixirs. Then simply keep the jar in direct sunlight for approximately twelve hours to allow the vibrations from the crystals to charge the water.

When the elixir is ready, take out the crystals and store the water tincture inside amber-colored glass bottles with an airtight seal. It will remain effective for one week. If you need the elixir to last longer, you can add fifty percent vodka or brandy to preserve it for up to a year or more. You can dilute the tincture for daily use by adding only seven drops of the pure elixir to a two-ounce glass dropper bottle filled with water and one-third brandy. Take seven drops of this tincture three times daily. For severe Root Chakra blockages, gradually increase the amount of pure elixir in your daily dosage bottle each week.

Aromatherapy

Essential oils are potent, natural medicines that can purify your Root Chakra. They are easily absorbed through the skin to help stimulate the body's natural abilities to restore the immune system and regenerate damaged body tissue.

The effects essential oil fragrances have on the brain are profound as well, and this aromatherapy helps balance brain activity, emotions, and hormone secretions.

It's best to use the highest quality essential oils of cedar wood, ginger, black pepper, cloves, and rosemary to treat Root Chakra imbalances. You can use them individually or in various combinations as you please.

Before you begin working with these oils, you must dilute them in a carrier oil – such as jojoba, almond or sesame oil – first, because they will irritate your skin if you apply them directly, without any dilution. Clove is the most potent of the oils mentioned above, and it should therefore be diluted the most; in your blend, use four times as much of your base carrier oil as you do of pure clove oil.

Take care to never bring these oils or oil blends near your eyes during use.

Once your blend is ready, you can massage your feet with it before you go to sleep at night. You can also rub it into your lower back, hips and thighs to target the Root Chakra area more effectively. It's particularly soothing to give yourself an oil massage twenty minutes before you take a bath because then the oils can penetrate more deeply into your relaxed muscles and circulate better throughout your body to stimulate healing.

For a more intensive treatment, you can find a local massage therapist who uses essential oils during acupressure sessions and specifically request the use of the above-mentioned oils during your session. Rubbing essential oils directly into the body's meridians and acupressure points provides the best results.

For pure aromatherapy purposes, you don't need to dilute these oils. In this case, you can simply carry around your pocket-sized oil bottle and inhale it as often as you like for a little healing refreshment throughout your day. At home, you can also use a cold air diffuser to release pure, healing scents directly into the air.

It's rare that anyone experiences negative side effects from essential oil use. If you do, however, avoid using other synthetic or petroleum-based fragrances and other personal care products on your body while you are undergoing essential oil treatments and aromatherapy. If you have a history of epilepsy or high blood pressure, consult your doctor before using essential oils. Anyone who is prone to skin allergies should begin by testing essential oils on the soles of their feet, and you can always dilute your oil blend with more vegetable oil to soothe the skin as needed.

Yoga Poses

Yoga postures stimulate all of the body's restorative processes and bring your mind, body, and spirit back into balance.

Some of the most effective yoga poses for cleansing and balancing your Root Chakra (and their names in Sanskrit) are:

Bridge pose (*setu bandha sarvangasana*),
Seated angle pose (*upavishta konasana*),
Standing mountain pose (*tadasana*), and
Standing forward bend pose (*uttanasana*)

You can easily do these poses at home, but if you have a history of major back problems or have had surgery around your abdomen, back, or legs, seek the direct instruction of an experienced yoga teacher to prevent injuries and consult with your doctor.

Tadasana (Standing Mountain Pose)

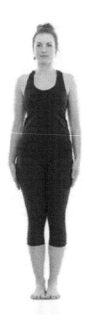

Place your feet together and let your arms hang down by your sides. Push both of your feet firmly into the ground to stand tall and proud, like a vast mountain range. Shift your weight slightly backward and then forward, until you find your center, and then distribute your weight evenly throughout your feet and toes. Imagine there is a straight rod that runs from the bottom of your heels and up through your legs and back until it reaches the back of your head. Lift your chest, bring your shoulder blades close together behind you and extend your arms straight down. Breathe normally and keep your thighs active for a strong stance.

Uttanasana (Standing Forward Bend Pose)

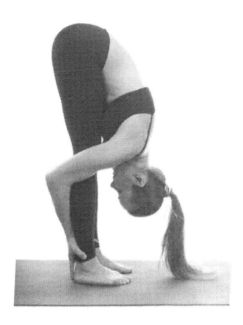

From your position in the first pose, lift both of your arms up into the air as high as you can. Inhale and look up at the sky. Then, as you exhale, let your arms lead your body to bend straight down to the floor and reach for your toes. It doesn't matter if you can't touch your toes - the important thing is to reach for them and pull the front of your chest and torso towards the floor while allowing your lower back to relax. Don't let your thigh muscles relax; keep them active to support your back as you try to hold this pose for at least one minute, breathing normally. Eventually, you can hold this pose for up to fifteen minutes for a deep release in the lower back and hamstrings. When you start to get really tired, slowly raise your torso back up by lifting from your thigh muscles.

Setu Bandha Sarvangasana (Bridge Pose)

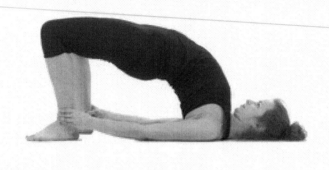

This pose is best done with a yoga block - unless you have lots of previous yoga experience.

Put both of your feet against a wall while lying on the floor, then move both feet to the ground just in front of the wall and push down with your feet to raise your pelvis in the air and place the yoga block underneath you. The block's job is to support your Root Chakra area five to six inches above the floor. You'll have to adjust yourself a little closer to the wall as needed so you can lift both legs up and push the soles of your feet slightly into the wall, keeping your legs straight. Use your hands to help support your lower back - as your shoulders remain on the floor - and lift your chest. Hold this pose only for a few minutes at first, and then put both feet down on the floor again to lift your buttocks up off the block, remove the block, and relax onto the floor.

Upavishta Konasana (Seated Angle Pose)

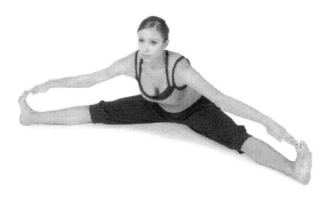

Seated on the ground, extend your legs straight out in front of you. Next, pull your right leg to the right as far as you can, then pull your left leg to the left as far as you can. You can use your hands to help support you in sitting up straight by placing them on the ground next to your hips. Keep your toes pointed straight up in the air and push your heels forward to keep your legs active as you sit. You can stretch your arms out and try to touch your toes, or you can stretch them out in front and place your hands on the floor. After a minute, you can push yourself forward on the floor a little to intensify the stretch as it becomes more comfortable. To come out of this pose, use your hands to help pull your legs together before getting up.

Reiki

Reiki is a powerful energy healing technique that's been passed directly from teachers to students over many years. The healer sends positive energy through their hands into the patient's body; such a healer can also remove energy blocks as well as any stored negative energy.

This treatment is deeply restorative for Root Chakra trauma, and you can also study Reiki and seek initiation yourself from an experienced teacher. After initiation, you'll be able to actively heal yourself with this positive energy.

When selecting a Reiki teacher or therapist, it's very important to check his or hers credentials and references because not all Reiki practitioners are of the same quality.

Dowsing

Dowsing is a special technique that relies on a pendulum made of crystal or other precious metals that helps to access the deeper subconscious wisdom and direct the healing abilities of the user.

Training is necessary in order to use it well. The professional healer can use pendulum dowsing to clear individual Chakras, pinpoint areas that need treatment in the body, and determine which types of treatments will be the most effective for each individual.

Like Reiki, dowsing treatments require initial oversight from an experienced healing professional, but you can learn how to use them for self-healing.

APPENDIX - A Brief Explanation of The 7 Chakras

The First Chakra, the Root (or Base), is deep, rich red. It is literally located at the base of the spine. The Universal Life Force energy (chi) enters the body here, through the Root Chakra, and moves upward.

This Chakra roots us to the Earth to support our survival and provide grounding. When the First Chakra is in balance, we feel secure and aware at the most basic level. We can give and receive love and provide for all our body's physical needs - food, shelter, clothing, and survival.

Out of balance, this Chakra could express its condition with issues such as being ungrounded, fear of moving forward in life, general anxiety, and addiction. Physically, the body might respond with pain, feel mentally spacey, have colitis, diarrhea, or menopausal symptoms.

The Second Chakra is called the Sacral; it connects to the sacrum, located just below the navel, behind the genitals. Its color is orange-red. It is the lower emotional aspect addressing earthly and bodily emotions.

Here, the Sacral drives the sensual urges and sexuality. Promiscuity and lack of sex drive are both imbalances of the Second Chakra. This is also the home of the "gut feeling," where we admit we know things but have no reason for our certainty. That feeling is the result of the dual aspect of spiritual energies coming from the Crown Chakra and interacting with the base energies of our grounding with Earth in the Root Chakra. We are naturally balanced here, expanding recognition and acceptance of our dual nature, allowing us to enjoy a strong spiritual and physical mindset.

This is the physical home of sacred sex - the orgasm and sexuality - as well as the spiritual home of all impressions and visualizations. An imbalance here endangers fertility and engenders depression. When they can't deal with feelings of guilt and humiliation, people often store those negative feelings here.. Holding all of that negative emotion here is damaging, blocking progression of energy to the next Chakra and, worse, creating fear and disgust of ourselves.

Balance brings great reward: this is the seat of Visualization, a tool for manifesting the mind's dreams and desires and bringing them onto the earthly plane – that is, establishing any dream in the here and now. It is a place of unusual empowerment for those who wish to meditate or focus on seeking their inner self, as well as for those who desire integration with the Universal Life Force Energy.

The Third Chakra, following the progression of the prism or rainbow, shines a clear yellow or the yellow-green purity of new growth plant shoots. It is found at the solar plexus, just above the naval. Universal Life Energy flows strongest into this Chakra, affecting our feelings about everything. Health and happiness are the rewards of balancing this Chakra.

The Chakra affects two divergent aspects of the mind: depending upon the state of the Third Chakra, the mind can be focused on maintaining willpower or it can be lost to apathy. Since ideas and assimilation are controlled here, it is a manifest power center – or not – depending on your choices and actions.

An imbalance will result in fear and anger in your pursuits, but, when in balance, your confidence and purpose will shine the pure golden yellow of the Sun on your dreams and point to the road for success.

So it makes sense that, when your emotions are out of whack at home, in the workplace, with your kids, or in the world at large, this is the Chakra that will provide the doorway to balance.

The Fourth Chakra is a fresh, bright green or sometimes a rose red. It is found at the physical heart and its balance is essential for healing. It is the seat of love, respect, and joy in us - as well as surrender.

As the Center of all Chakras, it is also the connection through which all energy flows in either direction. Here earthly energies are converting to the Spiritual as well as the reverse. Unconditional love and the desire to care for ourselves and others flow out from here. It is the seat of our empathetic nature and sympathy.

The Fifth Chakra, found at the throat, is the first of our spiritual centers, and it has no connection to our earthly plane. Resonating as the pure blue of lapis, it is a gateway to our intuition and psychic abilities – to seeing the invisible world. Our sense of self and the creation of our personal needs and desires are centered here. Professional capability or an excess of pride and blaming others are among the consequences of the Fifth Chakra's balance or imbalance.

The Sixth Chakra is well known as the Third Eye. Its color is the deep blue of indigo. Located in the center of our forehead, it is the place where we find our intuition. Psychic ability flows from here. The all-important mind-body connection can be accessed and strengthened here. Clairvoyance and the ability to generate great ideas for good or evil depend on the balance of this Chakra.

The Seventh Chakra sits as the top of our heads, where the fontanel was open in infancy. It is also the area enclosed by a sovereign crown, and became known as the Crown Chakra. Our ultimate spiritual connection and the integration of our physical, mental, emotional, and spiritual wholeness lie here in this center.

About The Author

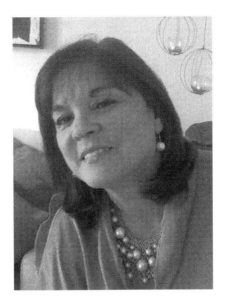

Mirtha Contreras was attracted to everything related to personal growth and spirituality for as long as she can remember. She began her professional training as a rebirther almost 20 years ago and went on to create her own Rebirthing School, where both her study of personal growth and career began to flourish. Mirtha's interest in how the emotional intertwines with the energetic grew over the years, and she went on to be trained as a teacher in Spiritual Response Therapy.

Over the years, Mirtha has helped hundreds of clients and students, using her skills as a Reiki Master, facilitator for the EMF Balancing Technique ®, Systemic Family Therapist (Family

Constellations), trained practitioner of The Reconnection (by Dr. Eric Pearl) and Reconnective Healing, and as facilitator of the Mindful Self-Awareness technique (AONC, by Dr. Javier Villegas). She has also appeared as an expert guest on numerous TV and radio shows.

Every step she has taken on her career path is driven by her enthusiasm to serve people who want to learn more about managing their emotional state and the energetic power needed to shift consciousness and harness personal strength.

Mirtha strives to help people become aware of their own inner power in order to increase their confidence as they recognize that we are all able to overcome any obstacle and achieve our goals, and she aims to do so with the best attitude and disposition. For Mirtha, witnessing these changes is the most fulfilling aspect of her work.

Made in the USA
Middletown, DE
18 January 2018